POSTPARTUM RECOVERY

How You Can Have A Better Postpartum
Recovery

Dr. Gracie Silver

TABLE OF CONTENTS

PRESENTATION

The moment you've been waiting for is finally here. Your little one is now a part of the outer world after months of caring for a developing baby inside your womb and exhausting hours of childbirth. Best wishes!
You just accomplished a really challenging and exquisite job. The shift from pregnancy to postpartum is about to happen, and it's likely that you'll feel worn out, sore, and a bit nervous. But what precisely can you anticipate following childbirth?
One of the most amazing things your body has ever accomplished is growing another human. You're probably eager to bring your new baby home after nine months of waiting. You'll be devoting a lot of your attention and energy in the upcoming weeks and months to but remember that you also need to take care of yourself, too.
It might have been simple or complex how you delivered it. You might have delivered your baby vaginally or via cesarean section (C-section). It's possible that you labor for a few hours or several days. Whatever the appearance of your delivery, your body has experienced trauma. Recovery will take some time.
You won't recuperate from giving birth in a matter of days. It may take months to fully heal from pregnancy

and childbirth. Feeling like yourself again may take longer than the 6–8 weeks when many women feel mostly recovered. You can have the impression that your body is against you throughout this period. Try not to lose your temper. Keep in mind that your body is unaware of your expectations and deadlines. Rest, healthy eating, and taking time for yourself are the finest things you can do for it.

It is also at this period that your hormones will be changing. You'll likely be more emotional and unable to think rationally. Again, allow yourself time for this to pass. Tell someone, nevertheless, if you ever consider harming your child or yourself. Or give the Suicide and Crisis Lifeline a call.
In the days and weeks after giving birth, your body and emotions will undergo significant changes. These are some of the most important things to anticipate both throughout the postpartum period and right after giving delivery.

Chapter 1

TIMELINE FOR POSTPARTUM HEALING

How Much Time Is The Postpartum Phase?

The first six weeks following childbirth are widely regarded as the postpartum recovery period, regardless of the method of delivery.
This does not imply that you will return to your pre-pregnancy state by magic at six weeks. Rather, this speaks of the physical recovery that occurs in your body following childbirth, known as postpartum healing. Growing and giving birth took more than a year. Rest easy knowing that you will feel like yourself far sooner than that, for the most part. You ought to be well on your road to recovery in a few months.

That is not to suggest that there won't be difficulties with postpartum healing. It is quite typical to have the impression that your body is not recovering as rapidly as you would like. Recall that you'll benefit more from resting your body and allowing it to heal completely. Even if you can simply manage to eat, sleep, and care for your infant, that is enough.

Throughout the first six weeks, be mindful of your body. Try to observe changes in your own body, even though

you'll be exhausted and preoccupied with your infant. As you heal, this is crucial.
As you start to feel better, resist the want to do more. Overdoing activities at this phase can impede your recuperation. Concentrate on feeding your body healthy meals, drinking lots of water (particularly if you're breastfeeding), and getting enough sleep.

If you had a C-section, you will have greater restrictions on what you may do in the days and weeks after birth. Driving and lifting anything heavier than your kid are two common no-nos. Your doctor will let you know when you can return to normal activities.

Here is more of what you can expect during your postpartum recovery.

How long does it take to heal after giving birth?

By the six-week mark, your vagina, perineum or C-section incision should be healed, and your uterus should be back to its normal size. Throughout those first weeks, you'll experience a lot of changes – from new levels of tiredness to hormone fluctuations. And you'll probably continue to see changes in your body and emotions after the initial six weeks of recovery. For example, if you developed varicose veins during pregnancy, it may take up to 12 weeks for them to fade or go away

Here's more of what to expect throughout your postpartum recovery.
How long does it take to heal from giving birth?
By six weeks, your vaginal, perineum, or C-section incision should be healed, and your uterus should have returned to normal. During the first few weeks, you'll notice a number of changes, from new levels of exhaustion to hormonal shifts. After the first six weeks of recovery, your body and emotions will most likely continue to alter. For instance, if you had varicose veins during pregnancy, it could take up to 12 weeks for them to diminish or disappear

Your postpartum body: How will your body feel and change after giving birth?

Changes in postpartum hormones
Hormones are chemical messengers that inform your body what to do and when. During pregnancy, your hormones shift to assist your developing baby and prepare your body for childbirth. After giving birth, your hormones are on a new mission to assist you in healing, bonding with your baby, and, if desired, breastfeeding.
The first postpartum hormonal changes your body will experience are:
When you birth your baby and placenta, your estrogen and progesterone levels drop.
Oxytocin, often known as the bonding hormone, surges, contributing to the strong maternal impulse you will experience.

Prolactin levels rise to signal milk production.

Chapter 2

BLEEDING AND VIRGINIA DELIVERY

As your uterus sheds the thick lining it had throughout your pregnancy, you'll notice some vaginal bleeding and discharge, known as lochia. Even if you had a cesarean (C-section), you will have bleeding and discharge. It is usual to experience vaginal bleeding after giving birth, even if you had a C-section. This is your body's technique of removing the excess blood and tissue utilized to grow and nurture your kid. Expect it to be heavier at first (up to 10 days), but then taper down. Light bleeding and spotting can remain for up to six weeks following birth. It is critical that you exclusively use sanitary pads throughout this period. Using tampons can introduce bacteria and cause infection. Also, expect to pass some clots, especially in the first week. If the clots are larger than a quarter, you should consult your doctor.

Lochia will appear brilliant red for a day or two before gradually changing to pink, then light brown or light yellow. Bleeding and discharge will be most severe in the first few days following birth, but will gradually subside. Lochia typically lasts 4-6 weeks, with the discharge gradually decreasing.

What amount of bleeding is too much?

Early on, it may appear that you are bleeding profusely, akin to having a very heavy period. This is quite normal, but there are a few warning signals to look for.

What Amount Of Bleeding Is Too Much?

Early on, it may appear that you are bleeding heavily, akin to having a very heavy period. This is quite normal, but there are a few warning signals to look for.

If you are soaking through one pad each hour for more than two hours, contact the nurse line or your care provider immediately. Also, if you continue to have bloody discharge or blood clots for more than four weeks, contact your healthcare physician.

Increased bleeding after your lochia begins to subside could indicate that you're overdoing it and should rest more. Seeing recurrent clots could indicate that your uterus is having difficulty returning to its pre-pregnancy size. In either scenario, it is always preferable to call.

When should you expect your first postpartum period?

Several factors can influence when you start your period after giving birth. One of the most important elements is if you opted to breastfeed your baby and if your breastmilk is their exclusive source of nutrition. Those who do not breastfeed may have their period sooner than those who do - anywhere from four weeks to three months after giving birth. Some breastfeeders may experience their period around the same time, but many may not until they have begun to wean or have stopped breastfeeding totally.

Chapter 3

THE POSTPARTUM JOURNEY

After delivery you are going to experience some discomfort. Here are some discomforts you might experience after delivery .

Vaginal and perineal discomfort

The strain of labor will leave your vagina and perineum (the area between your vagina and rectum) swollen and aching.

The perineum is the area between the vagina and the anus. Often, this region tears during birthing. Other times, your doctor may need to make a minor cut in this area to widen your vagina before birthing. Even if neither of these events occurred during your vaginal birth, your perineum will be painful and probably swollen thereafter. You may experience soreness in this location for several weeks. While you heal, sitting on an ice pack for 10 minutes several times each day will help relieve pain. This is very beneficial after going to the bathroom. During the first week postpartum, use a spray bottle to clean the perineum with warm water after using the restroom. Notify your doctor if your perineum area continues to be uncomfortable or if you notice any signs of infection.

Contractions or aches after birth

Breastfeeding may make you more aware of postpartum aches. Breastfeeding helps your body to release oxytocin, which induces uterine contractions. Contractions after birth, too Contractions or aches after birth
Contractions after birth, often known as after-birth pains, can be difficult at times, but they are nothing compared to what you may have felt during labor. Actually, contractions after birth are a healthy sign. After-birth contractions help to minimize uterine bleeding and shrink the uterus back to its pre-baby size.

Breastfeeding may make you more aware of postpartum aches. Breastfeeding helps your body to release oxytocin, which induces uterine contractions. After-birth pains can be difficult at times, but they are nothing compared to what you may have felt during labor. Actually, contractions after birth are a healthy sign. After-birth contractions help to minimize uterine bleeding and shrink the uterus back to its pre-baby size. Breastfeeding may make you more aware of postpartum aches. Breastfeeding helps your body to release oxytocin, which induces uterine contractions.

Sore breasts

Your breasts have changed since the start of your pregnancy. The next dramatic shift will occur about the third or fourth day after giving birth, when your breasts

begin to fill with milk. Your breasts may get engorged and feel stiff, puffy, and painful.
Sore nipples and breasts are common during the first few days of nursing. If the ache lasts more than a few days, the infant may not be latching properly. Try a different position or get advice from a lactation professional. Do this before your nipples develop painful cracks that could interfere with breastfeeding.

The American Academy of Family Physicians (AAFP) recommends that all babies, with few exceptions, be breastfed or given expressed human milk exclusively for the first six months of life. Breastfeeding should continue with the inclusion of complementary foods during the second half of the first year. However, not all mothers are able to breastfeed for a variety of reasons, and formula is fine in those cases.

Whether or not you breastfeed, the initial tightness and pain will subside. However, if you decide to breastfeed, your breasts will normally feel full before you feed or pump them. If your next session is late, you may feel even more painful and heavy.
Blood flow to your nipples rises throughout your pregnancy, so you've probably been experiencing soreness for a few months. However, the first several days after giving birth increase the blood flow, making them especially sensitive. Naturally, choosing to breastfeed will have an effect as well.

It is normal for you to experience some pain while your baby learns how to correctly latch on to your breast. However, as the infant develops a good latch, this should subside. A little discomfort while the baby settles into a pattern is natural, but having continual pain throughout your feeding is not.
If you experience breastfeeding difficulties, a lactation consultant can be of great assistance - and you can request one right away in the hospital.

Muscles ache

You've just performed the mother of all exercises, therefore it's normal to feel muscle stiffness throughout your body after birth. And you may feel the impact of your efforts for a few days.

You should expect to be very sore anyplace you have a lot of stress during labor, such as your arms, neck, or jaw.

Water retention.

You may be eager for the swelling you saw during your pregnancy to subside. However, it won't be for a while. Also known as postpartum edema (swelling), your body will continue to retain water due to an increase in a hormone called progesterone. You may experience swelling in your hands, legs, or feet. It should not persist more than a week after birth. If it does, or if it appears to worsen over time, notify your doctor.

Weight Loss

If you expected to lose weight right away after having your kid, you were most likely disappointed. No mother is so fortunate, despite what you read in the newspapers. You should anticipate to lose 6-12 pounds (depending on your baby's size) during the birth. After that, your weight loss will slow down dramatically. Depending on how much weight you acquired during pregnancy (the average is 25-35 pounds), losing the baby weight could take several months. For many women, nursing appears to aid in weight loss. Other mothers do not see weight reduction during nursing. Try to maintain consistent nutrition while breastfeeding, and don't be discouraged if losing weight takes longer than you expected.

Tiredness

Fatigue is a perfectly normal postpartum symptom. Again, your body has just been through (and is still going through) a lot, so get as much rest as you can. Many health-care specialists encourage sleeping whenever your baby does. The most essential thing right now is the health of you and your child. Eating well and staying hydrated will also help you regain and sustain your energy levels over time.

Night Sweats

Postpartum night sweats are often caused by hormonal changes. They can be uncomfortable, but they are nothing to be concerned about. Just make sure to drink plenty of water and stay cool. Night sweats should stop in a few weeks.

Lower belly ache near the incision (if you had a C-section)

After a C-section, you will have discomfort and tenderness on and near your incision, especially in the first few days and weeks after recovery.
You will have abdominal pain as your uterus shrinks back to its natural size and shape. These pains are known as "afterpains." Most of these pains will be faint, but a few will be intense. You may experience more of these pains while breastfeeding your baby. Breastfeeding triggers a hormone in your body that causes the uterus to contract (tighten). For many women, applying heat to the area relieves pain. Consider using a hot water bottle or heating pad. Your abdominal ache should subside with time.
If these pains worsen or do not subside, you should contact your doctor

Recovery Timeline for C-sections

The postpartum healing period following a C-section is typically lengthier than for a vaginal birth. You will most likely spend an extra day in the hospital, and you will be restricted from bending and lifting. You may also be given pain medicine to take for one to two weeks following delivery.

Before you leave, you will receive full instructions on how to care for your incision and aid healing. Your incision should be healed in about six weeks after giving birth.

How to care for your C-section incision

When caring for your incision, be as gentle as possible while keeping it clean and dry. This may include cleaning your incision with mild soap once or twice daily. Run soap and water over it in the shower, or gently scrub it with a washcloth or bath sponge.

Remove extra water with a clean towel before air drying the remainder.

Wearing gauze bandages to absorb drainage and protect your clothes, and replacing the gauze every day or when it gets wet

How your mood, attitude, and emotions may change following childbirth

Having a new baby can bring a variety of feelings with it. Of course, it will be lovely and wonderful, but it will also place new demands on your time and energy.

Chapter 4

SOME CHANGES TO EXPERIENCE DURING POSTPARTUM

Baby Blues– You're highly likely to get some baby blues. After the joy and beauty of delivery, experiencing periods of depression, anxiety, or irritability can be unexpected and unsettling. But this isn't just typical; it's extremely common.

You're overjoyed to be bringing your baby home. The following minute, however, you are depressed. It can be confusing, particularly for new mothers. Know that many mothers (70-80%) experience sadness in the first few weeks after having a baby. Hormonal fluctuations create what is frequently referred to as the "baby blues". There is nothing to be ashamed of. In fact, confiding in a friend or family member can help you feel better. If you have these feelings for more than a few weeks or are unable to function as a result, you may have postpartum depression. Postpartum depression is more severe than the baby blues.

If you have significant emotions of depression or hopelessness, or you have thoughts of harming yourself or others, you should call your doctor immediately.

The baby blues may also cause insomnia or overwhelming feelings at times. However, they typically go away on their own within two weeks.

During this time, you should be especially gentle with yourself. It can be beneficial to talk about your feelings with your partner or loved ones. Share how you're feeling so that they can support you and guide you through this.

If your baby blues linger longer than two weeks or your symptoms worsen, contact your healthcare professional. You may be experiencing postpartum depression.

your interest in sex can decline.

There are various reasons why you may not want to be intimate with your partner after giving birth. You're exhausted and devoting a lot of time and energy to being a wonderful parent. Your body may still be recovering or undergoing hormonal changes.

Talking about what you're feeling with your spouse can help them better understand you. Furthermore, knowing when sex is considered safe again is critical for creating realistic expectations for yourself and your partner.

How Long After Delivery Can I Start Having Sex?

Around six weeks after giving birth, you can start having sex if you feel comfortable and your care provider approves. Remember that hormonal shifts might make your vagina feel dry and painful, especially if you're breastfeeding. Using a personal lubricant will reduce discomfort.

It is also possible to become pregnant during the postpartum period, even if you are breastfeeding and haven't started your period yet. It's difficult to predict when ovulation will return after having birth, so wear protection. Your postpartum visit is an excellent opportunity to discuss birth control options.

You might notice changes in your relationship with your partner.

You and your partner are certainly aware that your relationship will alter as a result of your baby's birth, yet it may still surprise you. It's quite natural. Both of your lives have changed, and it will take some time to adjust. Open and honest communication will be your most valuable weapon as you adjust to your new life as parents.

POINTS TO NOTE:

Pay attention to your body after childbirth. If something doesn't look right, it probably isn't. Soreness is to be expected during postpartum healing, but excessive discomfort could indicate a major problem. Don't be so focused on caring for your infant that you neglect your own health.

Just because you survived childbirth does not mean you are immune to health concerns. There are life-threatening complications from labor that can occur days or weeks after delivery.

Postpartum hemorrhage is uncommon but can occur. If your postpartum bleeding is filling more than one pad each hour, you should call your doctor right once. Without treatment, postpartum bleeding can be fatal. Severe and persistent headaches can indicate an underlying condition, particularly when combined with high blood pressure. You could be in danger of suffering a stroke.

Deep vein thrombosis (a blood clot in a deep vein) is a relatively uncommon issue (1 in every 1,000 pregnancies) that can develop during or after pregnancy. Symptoms include leg soreness or the sensation of having a strained muscle. Your leg may also feel red and hot to touch. Untreated, these clots can break free and migrate to your lungs. This can have serious consequences.

Postpartum preeclampsia is an uncommon condition that can develop within 48 hours of childbirth or up to six weeks later. It is comparable to preeclampsia (also known as toxemia), which can develop while pregnant.

Both preeclampsia and postpartum preeclampsia cause blood vessels to constrict (shrink). This causes high blood pressure and distresses your internal organs.

Unless you are monitoring your blood pressure, you may not notice any evident symptoms. When you do experience symptoms, they may include a strong headache, swelling in your hands and feet, impaired vision, pain in your upper right side, and abrupt weight gain. If you suspect you may have postpartum preeclampsia, call your doctor right away. When you are recovering from birth, it is best to err on the side of caution if you suspect that something is wrong with you or the baby. You should anticipate to feel some soreness as you recuperate. You shouldn't start to feel worse.

- In general, if you experience any of the following postpartum symptoms, contact your doctor.
- Heavy vaginal bleeding that soaks more than one pad each hour or vaginal bleeding that grows every day rather than decreasing
- Passing huge clots (more than a fourth)
- Chills and/or a temperature that exceeds 100.4°F
- Fainting or dizziness.
- Changes in your vision or a severe headache that persists
- Painful or difficult urination
- Vaginal discharge with a strong smell

- Heart palpitations, chest pain, or trouble breathing
- Vomiting
- The C-section or episiotomy incision is red, weepy (with pus), or swollen.
- New or worsening abdominal discomfort (lower belly)
- Sore, red, and burning breasts
- Pain in your legs with redness and swelling

Chapter 5

POSTPARTUM ESSENTIALS: WHAT YOU WILL NEED ON HANDS WHILE RECOVERING

Throughout your hospital stay, your care team will ensure that you have all you need to begin the postpartum healing process. (They may even send you home with a few items.) However, there are a few postpartum requirements you should have at home for when you return from the hospital.

- **Pain relieving medication**- Acetaminophen (Tylenol) and ibuprofen (Advil) are both pain relievers. Your doctor may even suggest rotating between the two medications during the first few days of recovery. Just be sure to follow their advice and ask any questions you may have. If you had a C-section, your doctor may have prescribed pain medicine during the first several weeks after delivery.

- **Belly Bands**-Belly bands provide gentle compression to assist relieve aches and pains as you heal. Bands wrap across your abdomen, from hips to ribs. Some women find that wearing a band alleviates back pain, supports their pregnancy-stretched core muscles, and relieves pressure on their C-section incisions. If you had a C-section, the hospital may have given you a postpartum belly band.

- **Absorbent maxi pads**-Tampons will be off limits until you have fully recovered, so you'll need comfortable yet absorbent maxi pads for the bleeding and discharge you'll experience.

- **100% cotton underwear** – Cotton is light and wicks away moisture. Because you'll be bleeding on and off for several weeks, and more strongly at first, choose underwear that you're willing to throw away if it gets soiled. You can also get disposable cotton underwear, identical to what the hospital will supply for you. (Tip: Request a few extra pairs of disposable underwear from the hospital. Many individuals find them really comfortable, especially in the first few days after having a baby.

- **Ice packs** – Ice packs in many forms are an excellent approach to relieve pain and inflammation. There are even wearable ice pads for the perineal and vaginal areas. But the traditional ice pack wrapped in a towel will still work wonders. Ice packs can help relieve pain from painful or engorged breasts.

- **Peri rinse bottle –As** your vagina and perineum heal, use a peri bottle or spray bottle full of warm water to aid healing and protect any sutures. Warm water is pleasant and allows you to gently rinse your perineal area after going to the bathroom. You will be given a peri bottle to take home from the hospital.

- **Sitz bath** –A sitz bath, in which you sit in warm, shallow water, can also help to relieve inflammation and clean your perineum. You can take a sitz bath in your bathtub or get a kit that includes a plastic bowl that attaches to your toilet. You can seat on water for 20 minutes three times daily .

- **Witch hazel pads** –Witch hazel pads are phenomenal for relieving postpartum hemorrhoids, but they can also aid with perineal soreness.

- **Hemorrhoid spray with lidocaine** –Lidocaine is a local anesthetic that is used in certain sprays. These sprays might provide quick, cooling relief from the discomfort and irritation caused by postpartum hemorrhoids.

- **Stool softener** –You may feel constipation in the weeks following childbirth. A stool softener can be a mild method to help things go along and reduce tension on your vaginal and perineal areas, especially if you have had stitches.

- **Nursing bras for day and night** –Nursing bras are meant to provide comfort and support without irritating sensitive places. They also include flaps that unzip, allowing your baby to feed without having to remove your bra. Even if you're not breastfeeding, a snug, comfy bra with solid support will work wonders. Wear bras without an underwire.

- **nipple creams** –There are specialized creams are the go-to treatment for aching, dry, or cracked nipples. They can be used whenever you're feeling uncomfortable. Many creams contain baby-safe components, so you don't need to wash them off before breastfeeding.

- **Nursing pads** – If you're breastfeeding, you're likely to encounter some milk leakage between feedings. Even if you are not breastfeeding, your breasts may leak a small amount of colostrum or milk early on. Nursing pads fit comfortably within your bra, absorbing leaks and preventing a wet shirt. You can choose between reusable and disposable pads. Both should be replaced during the day.

- **Heating pad** –The heating pad is a classic self-care tool. Resting against a source of mild, focused heat helps alleviate a variety of aches and pains, from the lower back to the breasts.

- **Help –**Your partner, family, and friends can be valuable resources while you heal. You have an essential task to do, so be willing to ask for and accept assistance with chores, meals, and anything else.